Adventure
to
Motherhood

the picture-story of pregnancy and childbirth

J. Allan Offen, M.D.

Assistant Professor of Obstetrics and Gynecology, University of
Miami School of Medicine; Attending Obstetrician and
Gynecologist, Jackson Memorial Hospital

Audio Visual Education Company of America, Inc.
Post Office Box 4008, Washington 15, D. C.

Preface

This book was written to tell a story, which is nearly as old as time itself. While the tale has retained all its wonderment and excitement throughout the centuries, modern obstetrics has modified the story, adding safety and a better chance of a happy ending to each retelling. It is my hope that this visual presentation of the true drama of pregnancy and childbirth will allay the fears, disprove the old-wives tales and answer the ever present questions of our young women and men, the mothers and fathers of tomorrow.

While it is impossible to credit all to whom credit is due, the contributions of some must be especially noted. I am very grateful to Dr. James H. Ferguson, Professor of Obstetrics-Gynecology, University of Miami School of Medicine and Dr. M. Edward Davis, Obstetrician and Gynecologist-in-chief, Chicago Lying-In Hospital for reading the manuscript and the supplements, and for their excellent suggestions.

I wish to express my deep and special gratitude to Commander Thomas B. Lebherz, M.C., U.S.N., U. S. Naval Hospital, Bethesda, Md., and Harry G. Zaritsky, Chief, Health Education, Audio Visual Division, National Naval Medical Center, Bethesda, Md., who have given freely of their judgment and experience to advise me on this work. Their assistance will have contributed in no small measure to whatever success this book may enjoy.

I am particularly grateful to the young couple in the book, Betsy and Jim; for without their cooperation this volume might not have been. I am also obligated to Hazel Corbin, R.N. and the Maternity Center Association for their permission to reproduce the slides of the Dickinson-Belskie childbirth models. The obstetric and nursing staff of the Jackson Memorial Hospital have earned my appreciation for their wholehearted cooperation in this undertaking. Jane Nichol, R.N., has been especially helpful. To Frank Zagarino and Phelps Schulke, go the credit for the colored pictures you are about to see.

The assistance and devotion of my office nurse, Mrs. Ethel Carroll, and my secretary, Mrs. Corinne Best, and the patient forebearance and encouragement of my wife and family cannot be overlooked.

In keeping with the tradition of dedicating books, this small volume is humbly and affectionately dedicated to mothers everywhere.

J. Allan Offen, M.D.

Miami, Florida.

Welcome to the greatest adventure in a woman's life.

Childbirth is natural and wonderful. Your doctor has been especially trained to guide you through this experience happily and help you deliver a healthy baby. Of course, he will need your cooperation in doing this and it is necessary that you follow his directions implicitly. There is a good reason for everything he does or instructs you to do.

You will find that your doctor is not only your physician and medical advisor, but also a trusted friend who is sincerely interested in you and available whenever you need him.

You may have many well-meaning relatives, friends or neighbors who are eager to give advice. Unfortunately, much of the time they are misinformed and their advice is poor. So, if you have a problem, if you are worried or troubled about anything, discuss it with your doctor; he can help you best.

The following pictures tell the story of one girl's adventure to motherhood. It could be you.

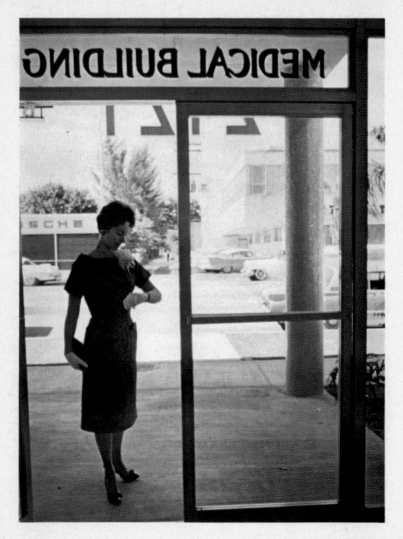

Three o'clock and a very important day; Betsy is on the way to keep her appointment with the doctor. During the past two months she has missed her menstrual periods, noticed some enlargement of her breasts and been aware of an increased bladder frequency. She hopefully suspects that she is pregnant.

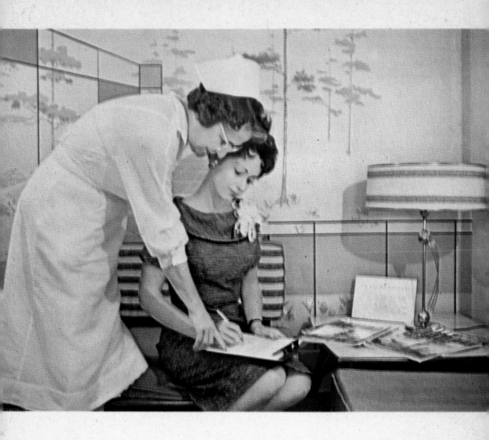

With the help of the office nurse, Betsy fills out a medical history form. A complete record is important so that the doctor may know what health problems she has had and can better evaluate her present state of health. Naturally this history is kept completely confidential.

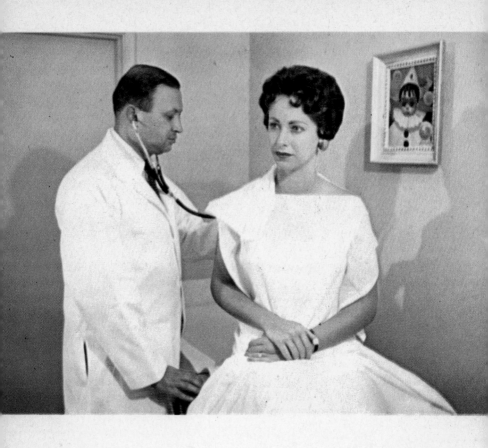

The doctor does a complete physical examination on Betsy after reviewing her medical history and asking questions about the way she feels.

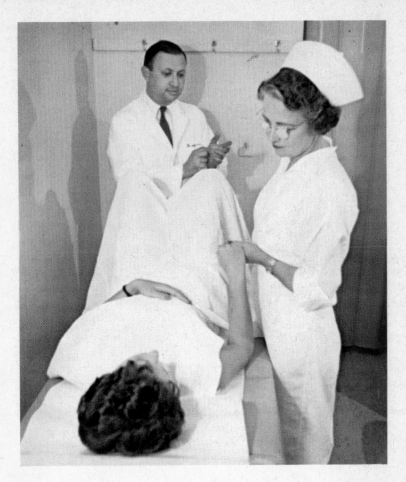

This includes a pelvic examination to determine whether her uterus has enlarged, for, if it has, the doctor usually can be quite sure that she is pregnant. "Well, Betsy," he finally informs her, "you're in excellent health and it certainly looks as though you're going to have a baby." While doing the pelvic examination, the doctor also obtains certain internal measurements of Betsy's bony pelvis and evaluates its contour. These give the doctor valuable information about the birth canal and what to expect in regard to childbearing.

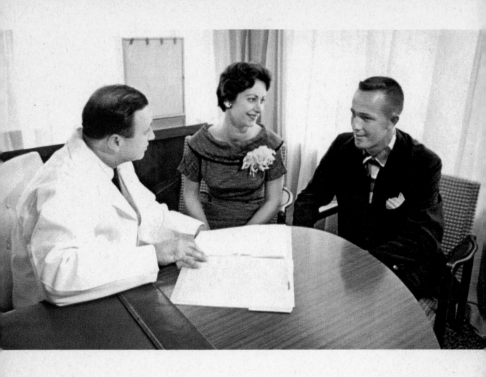

The doctor asks Jim, her husband, to join Betsy in the consultation room to discuss her pregnancy and what to expect. First, the doctor assures the young couple that the outlook for a good pregnancy and a pleasant delivery is excellent, provided they follow a few simple instructions.

"Pregnancy is a normal condition, Betsy, not an illness," the doctor says. "Most women feel better during pregnancy than almost any other time in their lives." The approximate date of delivery is calculated by taking the first days of Betsy's last menstrual period, counting backward three months, and then adding seven days.

"It is important during marriage to maintain mutual understanding and a warm relationship, especially during pregnancy. There is no need to alter sexual relations unless there is any bleeding, uterine cramps or difficulty. If you have any trouble call me."

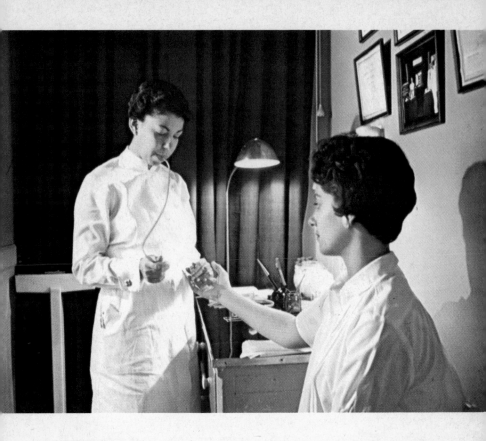

"I am going to order a series of laboratory tests which are important in pregnancy. These include a complete blood count, a serology test, determination of blood type, Rh type and a complete urinalysis."

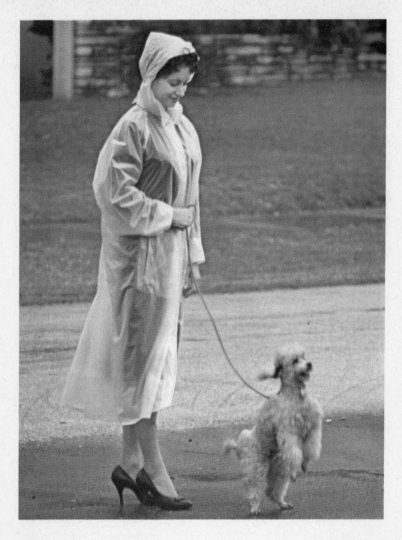

"Betsy, you should be able to maintain most of your normal activity. A moderate amount of exercise each day is essential—walking is particularly good. As a matter of fact, moderation in whatever you do is probably the best rule you could possibly follow during pregnancy."

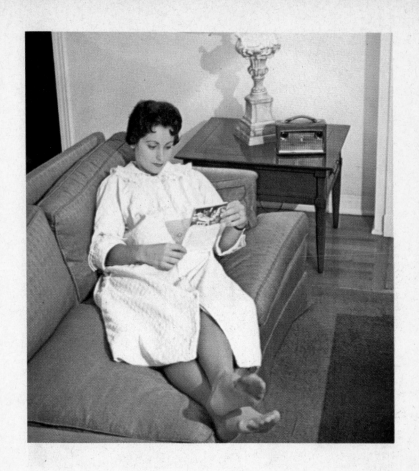

"Some rest each day is advisable, but you may continue to work for a while as long as you feel comfortable and do not get overtired. Obviously, exceedingly heavy work and fatigue should be avoided. You may bathe or shower during pregnancy but be careful not to slip or fall, especially during the late months."

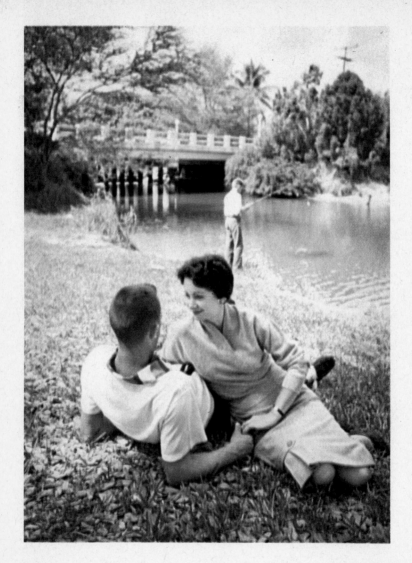

"When you take auto trips you ought to get out of the car frequently and walk for a few minutes. Long, tiresome automobile trips are probably inadvisable. If distant travel is necessary, plane or train are probably the best ways to go."

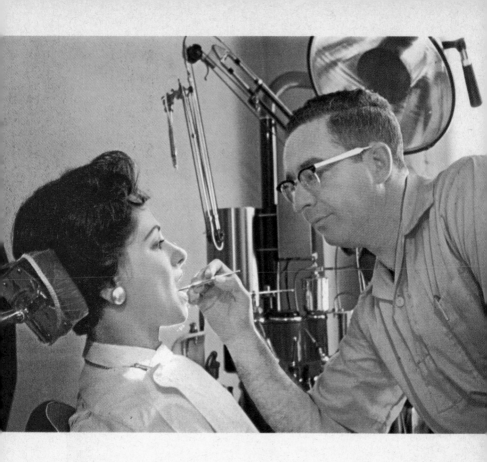

"Since oral hygiene is important during pregnancy, have your teeth checked by your dentist. If work is necessary, have it done in the early months when it will be easier for you."

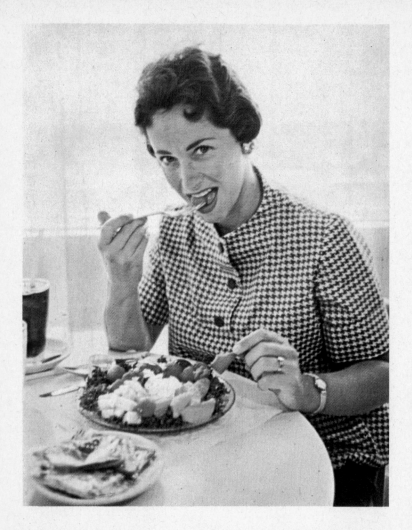

"Eat lean meats or fish, eggs, vegetables, cereals and milk every day to get the right amounts of protein, vitamins and minerals. The baby will get these important elements from your body and it is essential that you replace these daily to maintain your own health. A properly balanced diet for a moderately active woman should not exceed 2000 calories daily."

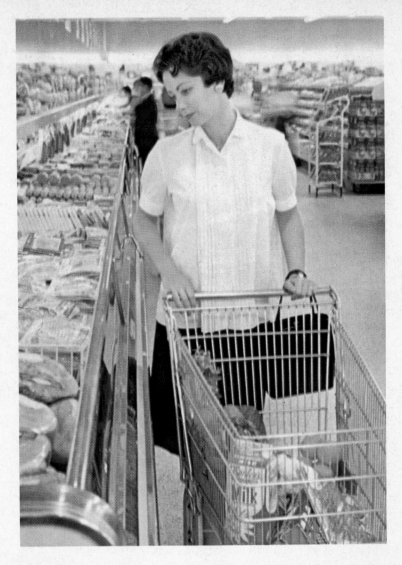

"Avoid all pastries, fried or fatty foods, cake, ice cream, nuts, salad dressings, rich desserts and soft drinks, but include ample fresh fruit each day."

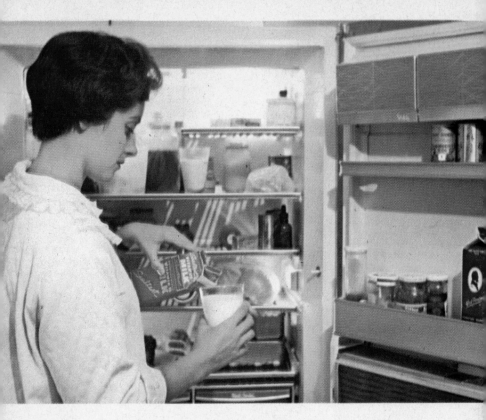

"If you gain too much weight, we may have to substitute skimmed milk or buttermilk for whole milk. You should have no trouble with your bowel function, if you exercise and maintain a proper diet with an adequate amount of bulk foods and roughage and drink five or six glasses of water every day."

"Salt restriction during pregnancy is also very important. Certain complications of pregnancy seem to be related to the retention of excess salt by the body and these usually can be prevented by limiting the amount of salt used in the diet. For the same reason baking soda should not be used. Potato chips, pretzels, olives, pickles, luncheon meats and other highly seasoned or salty foods should be avoided. Small amounts of salt can be used in cooking, but it is unwise to add salt at the table."

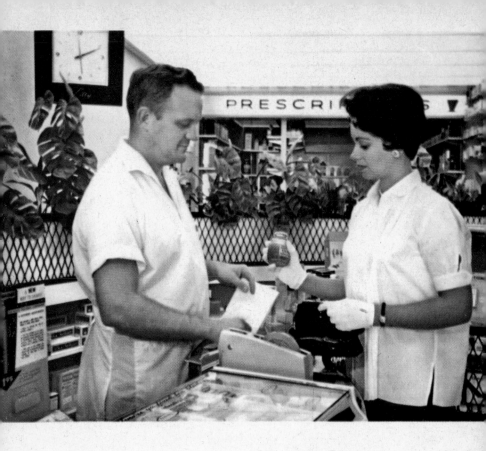

"You will need prenatal capsules to meet the added demand for iron, vitamins, minerals and trace elements, because the growing baby demands an excessive amount of these to manufacture blood. This will help prevent anemia during pregnancy."

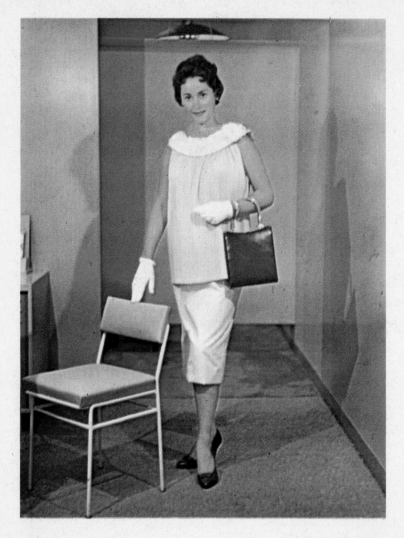

"Betsy, morale is one of the most important things during pregnancy and there is nothing like a nice appearance to give you a lift. Two or three stylish maternity dresses, an occasional trip to the beauty parlor, and an evening out once in a while, will work wonders and keep your spirits high."

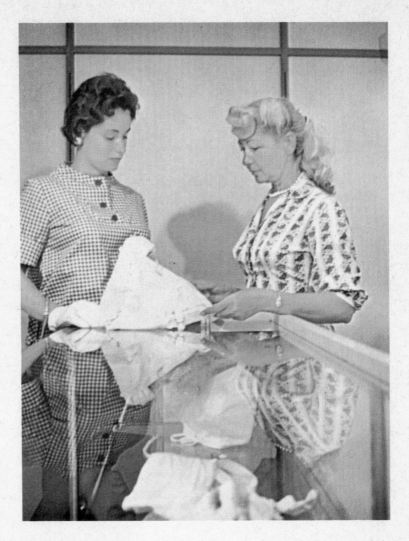

"A good maternity foundation garment and an uplift maternity bra may be very helpful in preventing a great deal of discomfort and backache and are really appreciated in the later months of pregnancy. Tight clothing or belts and garters that interfere with circulation should be avoided."

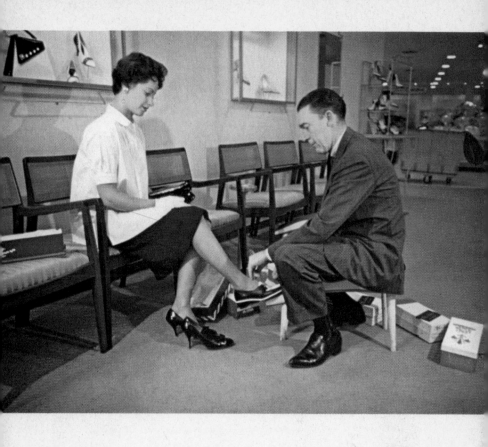

"Wear sensible shoes with a moderate or low heel and a good arch support. You will find that it will add to your comfort and safety."

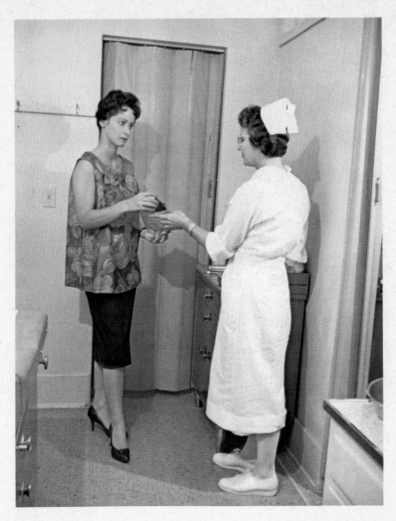

"On each visit bring a morning urine specimen to the office for examination. Frequent, regular visits to the doctor contribute to good prenatal care and the avoidance of complications. During the early months of pregnancy you will be seen at three-to-four week intervals. Later on, however, you will be seen much more frequently."

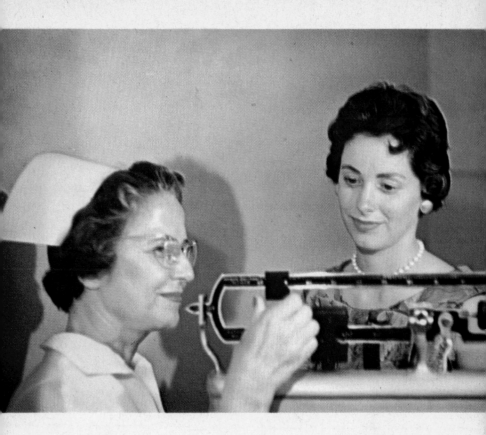

"You will be weighed each time and a careful record kept. During pregnancy there is a tendency to gain too much weight. You should not gain more than twenty pounds over the entire nine months. It is important to keep your monthly gain down to two pounds or less."

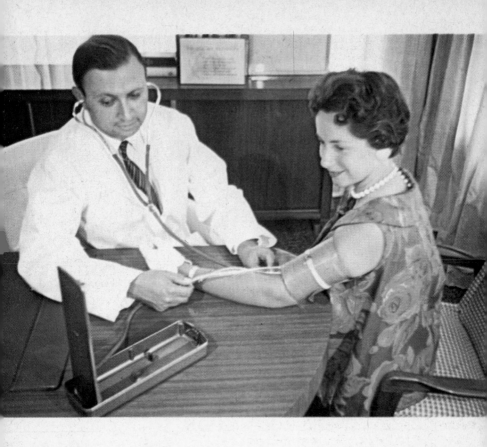

"At each appointment I or my nurse will take your blood pressure and during these visits, Betsy, feel free to discuss with me any problems or difficulties you may have."

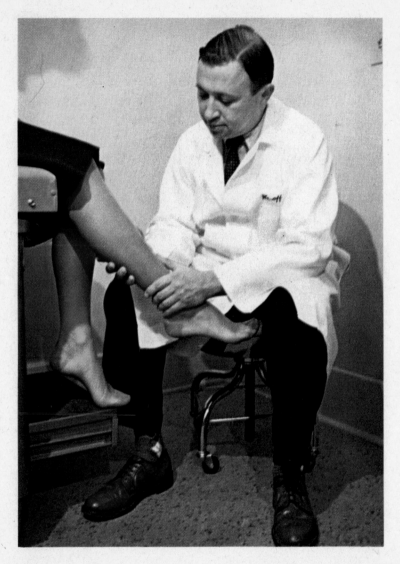

"Let me know if you notice any unusual swelling. As a precautionary measure your legs, hands and other likely areas will be checked each time."

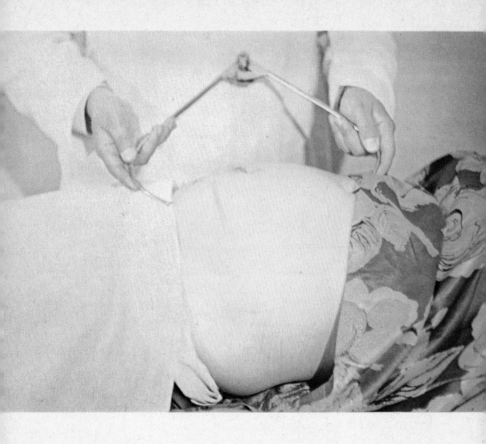

"The progress of your baby's growth will be followed by measuring the height of the uterus. Somewhere around the eighteenth or twentieth week you will probably feel life for the first time. Movement increases gradually as time goes on."

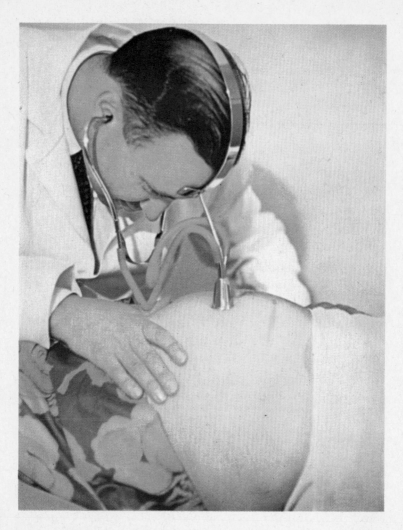

"The baby's heart beat can usually be heard at about twenty-four weeks. If the baby moves actively, I may not listen to it on each visit. However, during the last month of pregnancy listening for the heart sounds helps me to determine the position of the baby. To further evaluate the situation, an internal examination may be done in the last few weeks."

In many communities mothers- and fathers-to-be can attend classes in which the mechanics of pregnancy and childbirth are explained.

Using a projector and slides* the instructor covers a review of the anatomy and process of fertilization and implantation of the fertilized ovum in the uterus. The miraculous development of a baby from a single fertilized ovum is presented to show how the cells divide and form the body parts. The development and function of the umbilical cord and the placenta, which later becomes the "afterbirth", is also described. The natural mechanics of labor and delivery are discussed; the way the cervix thins out and then opens, allowing the baby to pass down through the birth canal with each contraction of the uterus; and the recognition of the onset of labor by the occurrence of regular, recurrent, rhythmic abdominal cramps or pain. These cramps may be associated with backache and if a hand is placed on the abdomen, the uterus can be felt to get very firm with each contraction.

In true labor the contractions usually become increasingly strong and the interval between contractions shorter. With the onset of labor, there may be some blood-streaked, mucoid vaginal discharge, known as "show." Early in labor, or sometimes even before labor begins, the membranes may rupture, releasing a gush of water from the vagina. Each patient is instructed to call the doctor if any of these circumstances occur.

*Slides reproduced with permission from the filmstrip "Having A Baby" published by the Maternity Center Association, New York City.

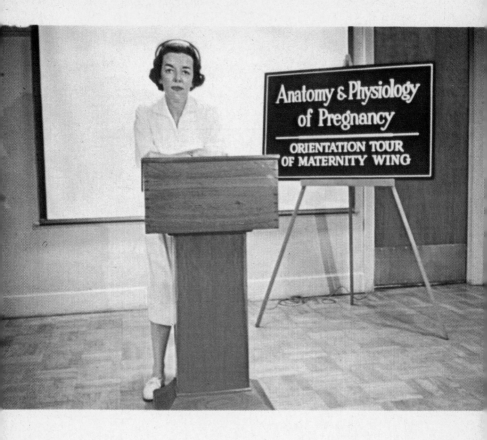

When all these natural processes have been thoroughly explained, each parent is given an opportunity to ask questions about any phase of human reproduction. Following this discussion period, the prospective parents are given a complete orientation of the hospital maternity wing either by conducted tour or the use of audio-visual aids.

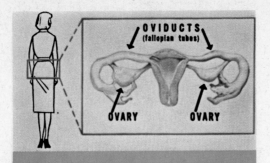

OVIDUCTS
(fallopian tubes)

OVARY   OVARY

This is where ova are produced.

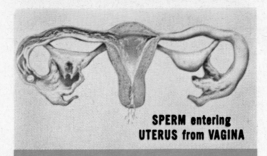

SPERM entering
UTERUS from VAGINA

Spermatozoa enter uterus and travel out
both oviducts to meet the ovum.

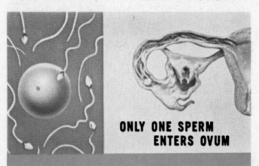

ONLY ONE SPERM
ENTERS OVUM

This is when a new life begins. A sperm
fertilizes an ovum in the oviduct.

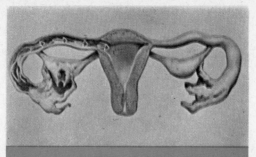

Fertilized ovum travels down oviduct to
uterus and finds a nesting place.

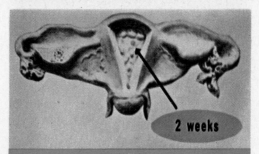

2 weeks

In two weeks—the baby is just a tiny dot
of cells, but all important parts of his body
are being formed.

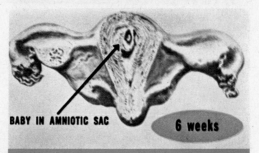

BABY IN AMNIOTIC SAC

6 weeks

Baby floats in amniotic sac which is
filled with fluid. His heart muscle has
begun to beat.

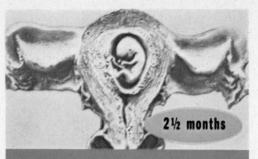

2½ months

The baby's body is well formed by now.
See umbilical cord and placenta.

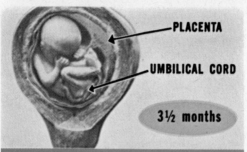

PLACENTA

UMBILICAL CORD

3½ months

The baby gets his food and oxygen,
and disposes of his waste through
placenta and umbilical cord.

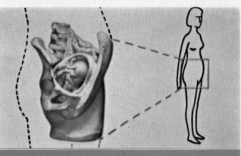

At 4½ months, baby fills the cradle of
his mother's pelvis. She may begin to
feel him moving.

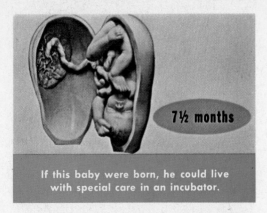

7½ months

If this baby were born, he could live with special care in an incubator.

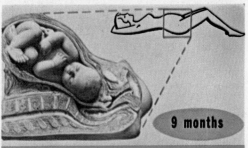

9 months

Ready to be born. Baby lies head downward in his mother's uterus.

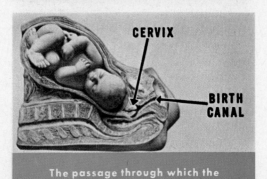

CERVIX

BIRTH CANAL

The passage through which the baby is born.

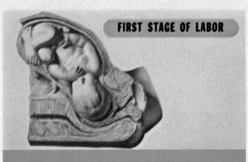

FIRST STAGE OF LABOR

The cervix is slowly opened by contractions of the uterus.

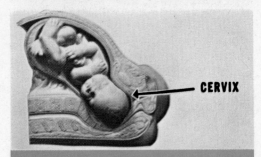

CERVIX

The cervix is thinned and pulled up.

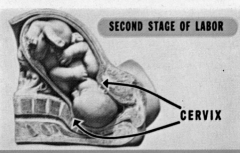

SECOND STAGE OF LABOR

CERVIX

The cervix is open. The mother, helped by the contractions, pushes the baby down the birth canal.

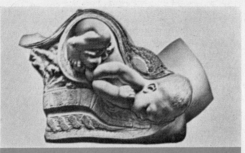

Baby's head begins to appear. Note moulding and turning of baby's head to fit the passage.

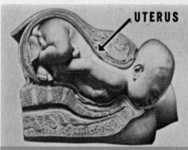

UTERUS

Just before birth. The top of the baby's head can be seen. Note how small the uterus has become.

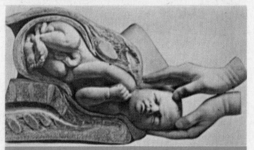

Birth! The doctor's hands guide the baby's head and shoulders as the baby is born.

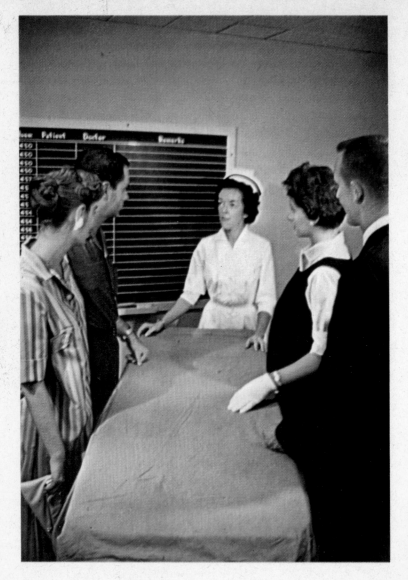

This orientation includes procedures for admitting the maternity
patient to the hospital when she is in labor.

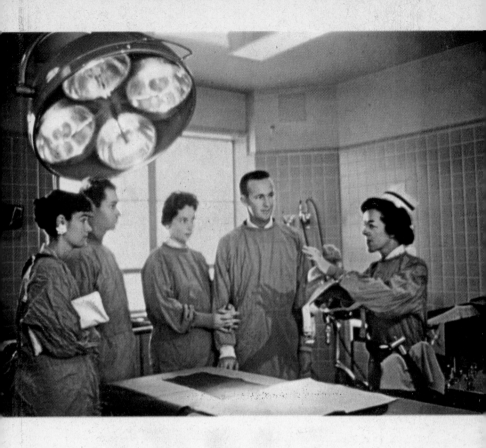

In communities where conducted tours are used, surgical gowns are provided to cover the visitors' street clothes. The group is shown through the labor, delivery and postpartum suites. In the delivery room the special tables, equipment and sterile techniques are demonstrated and explained.

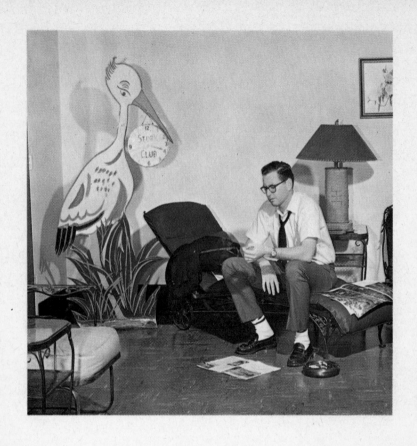

In the "Stork Club" an expectant father is awaiting in traditional fashion his new arrival.

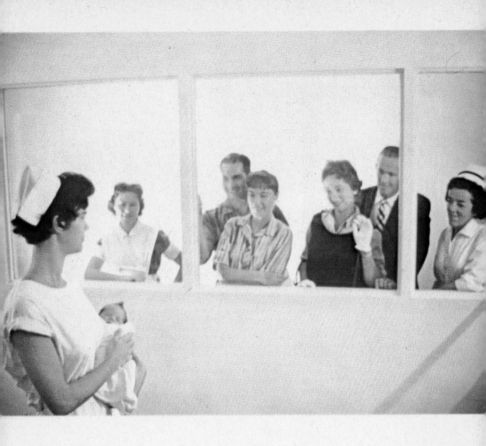

Finally they go to the nursery, the most exciting place of all, where the beautiful newborn babies can be observed through the plate glass windows and no one wants to leave.

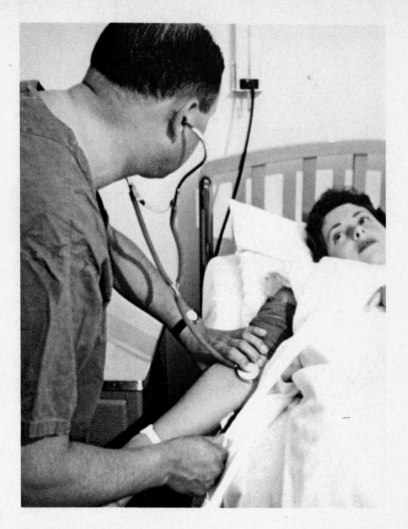

Now Betsy's ready to have her baby; not far from the date the doctor predicted many months ago. The contractions have been coming regularly and are now quite close together and the doctor has sent Betsy to the hospital. First she is given a perineal "prep" and a cleansing enema and is then put to bed with an identification band strapped around her wrist.

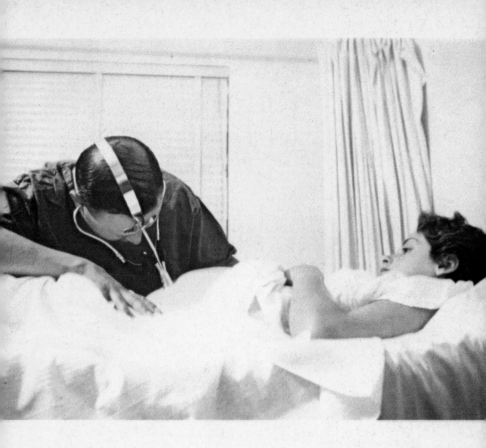

Shortly after her admission, the doctor checks Betsy's blood pressure and he assures her that she is progressing satisfactorily. Because of her prenatal education, Betsy has an understanding of what occurs during labor and delivery and has confidence in her doctor and the hospital staff. As a result she is completely relaxed.

The doctor listens to the baby's heart, and with his hand on the abdomen he is able to determine the force of the uterine contractions. From this and other examinations he can tell how labor is progressing.

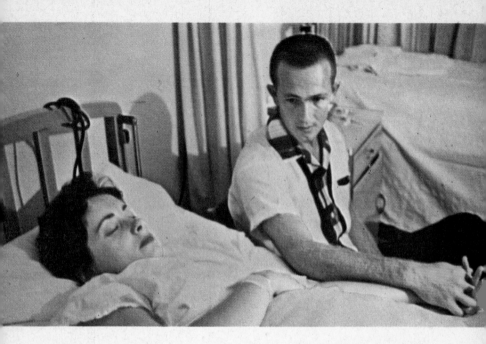

The doctor permits Jim to stay awhile with Betsy since she is still in early labor and there is no other patient in the room. Previously the doctor had told Betsy that if and when her uterine contractions caused her any discomfort he would use sedation to make her comfortable and at delivery he would give her an anesthetic. The particular sedation or anesthetic the doctor selects depends upon the patient, the duration of the pregnancy, the size of the baby and a number of other factors which he evaluates best at the time of labor. The choice of medication is left to the doctor who bases his decision on what is best for both mother and baby. Sometimes, there is a patient who prefers no sedation or anesthesia at all. In each case the doctor's objective is to effect a safe and pleasant labor and delivery.

When strong, muscular contractions of the uterus cause the mouth of the cervix to open completely and the baby is pushed down to the mouth of the birth canal, Betsy is taken to the delivery room. Because the baby is nearly ready to be delivered, she now is given an anesthetic.

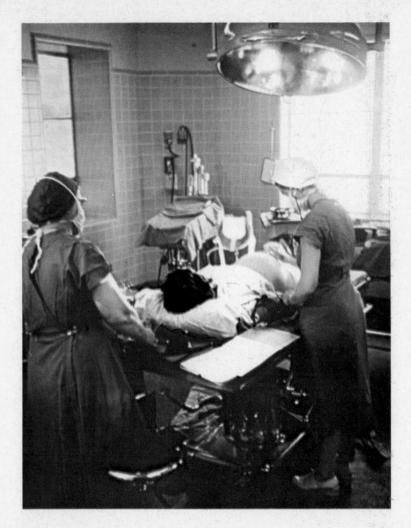

In the delivery room the baby's heart tones are checked frequently, in order to keep the doctor informed that everything is progressing satisfactorily. Soon, Betsy's legs are placed in stirrups to obtain a position for easy delivery of the baby. In preparation for this a thorough cleansing of the lower abdomen and perineum is carried out with an antiseptic solution.

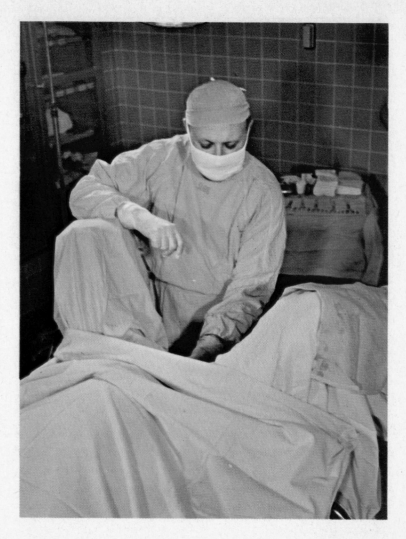

With the entire area covered with sterile drapes and leggings, the doctor makes an internal examination to determine the position of the baby's head. Forceps are frequently used to shorten labor and to prevent damage to both mother and baby. Of course, many babies are delivered without the use of forceps.

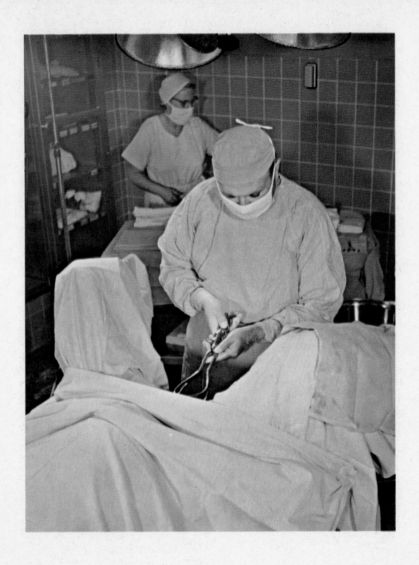

The forceps are held just as they are to be placed.

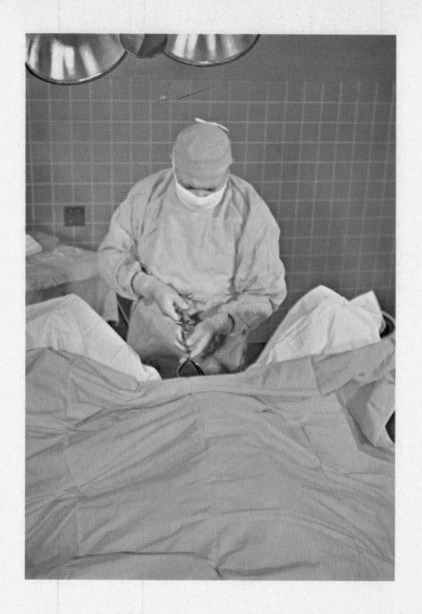

Then they are carefully applied and the delivery is gently started.

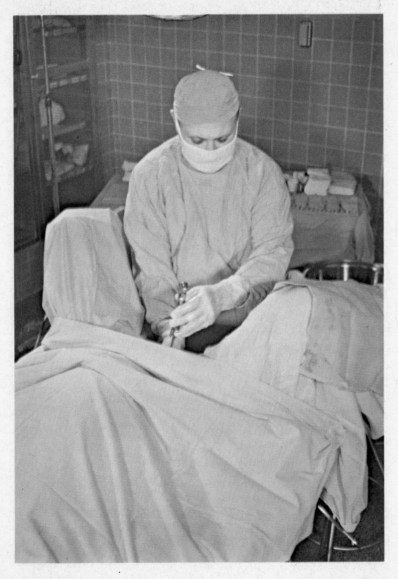

A small incision is made in the perineum to prevent any serious tears or lacerations. Of course, this is not felt because of anesthesia.

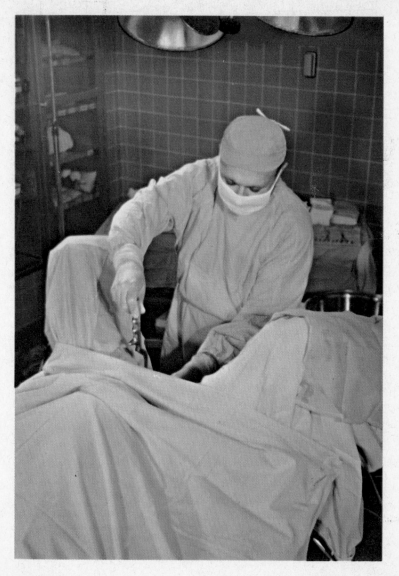

As the baby's head starts to come through the vulva the forceps are removed.

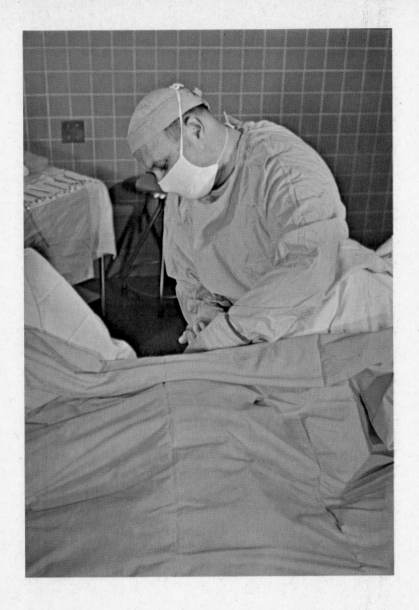

Now the head distends the perineum. The doctor gently guides it.

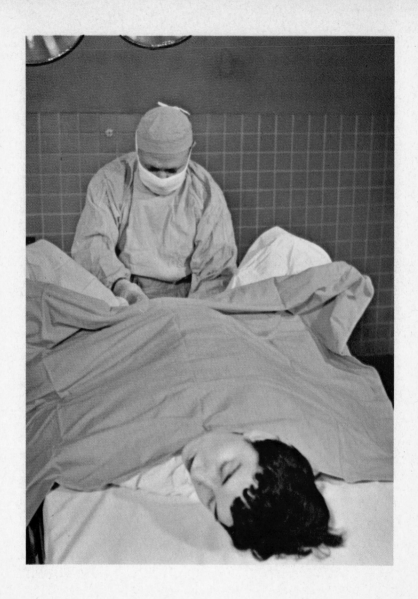

As the baby's head emerges,

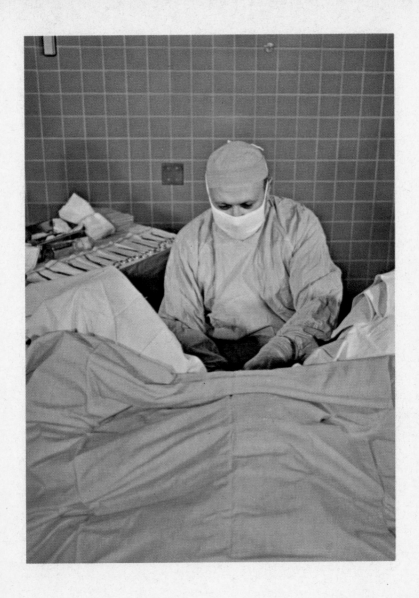

the doctor assists the natural muscular contractions of the uterus.

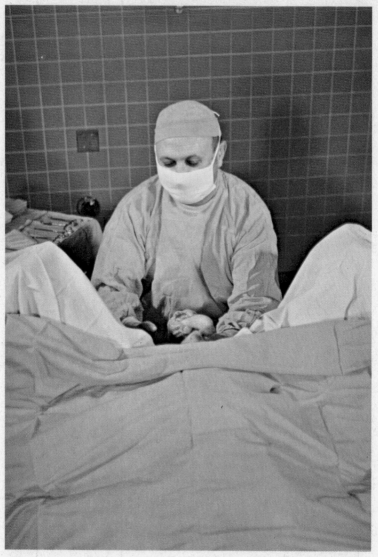

When the head delivers completely, the doctor removes the mucous secretions and fluids from the baby's nose and mouth.

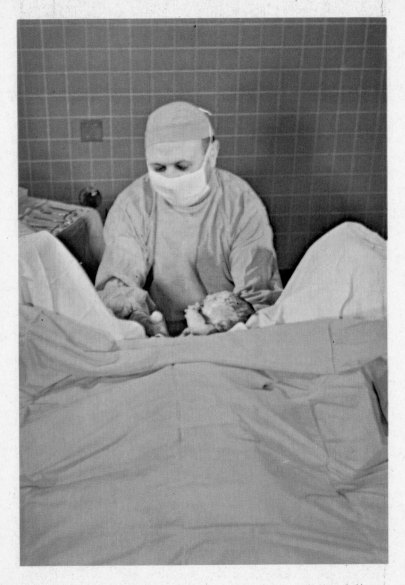

With the airway clear, the baby can breathe and the delivery continues to be conducted slowly with deliberation and care.

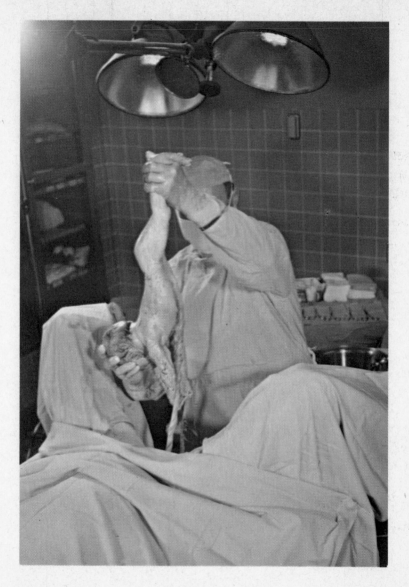

As the baby is completely delivered, the doctor firmly grasps the baby's feet in his hands and elevates them.

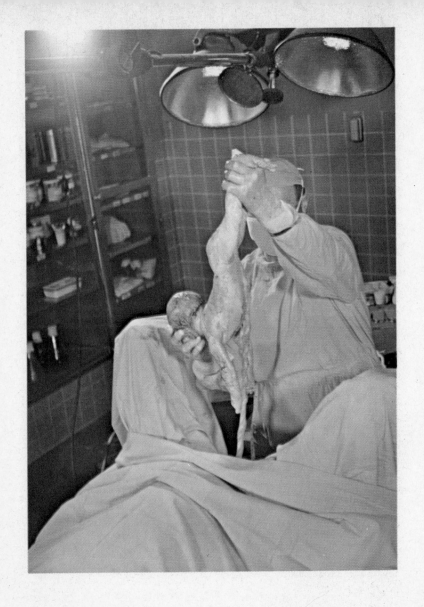

The baby is still attached to the mother by the umbilical cord.

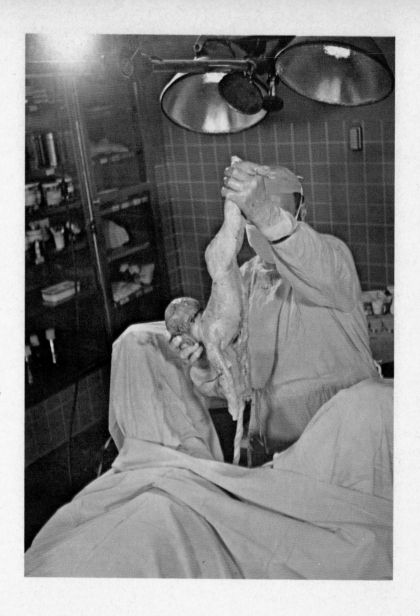

The infant usually begins to breathe and cry spontaneously.

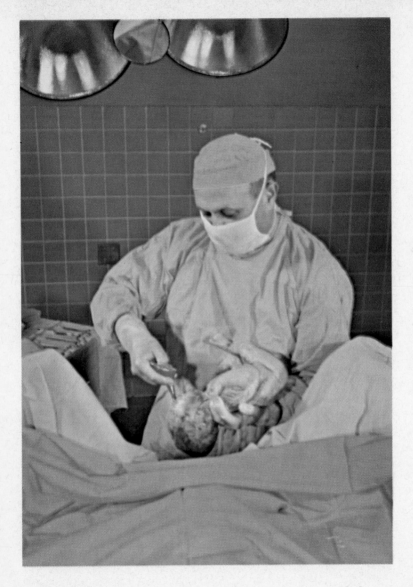

With the hand supporting the shoulders, the baby is turned over and held with the head lower than the body.

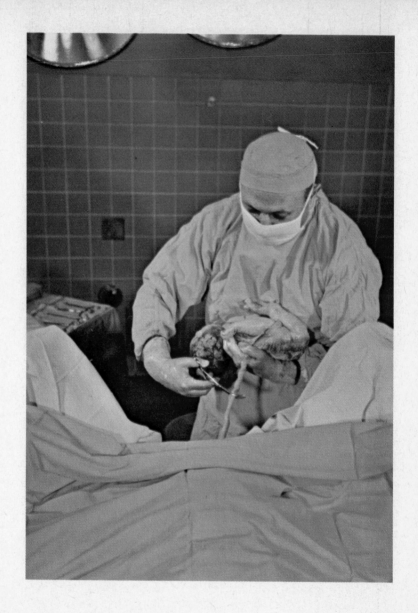

The cord is clamped and cut.

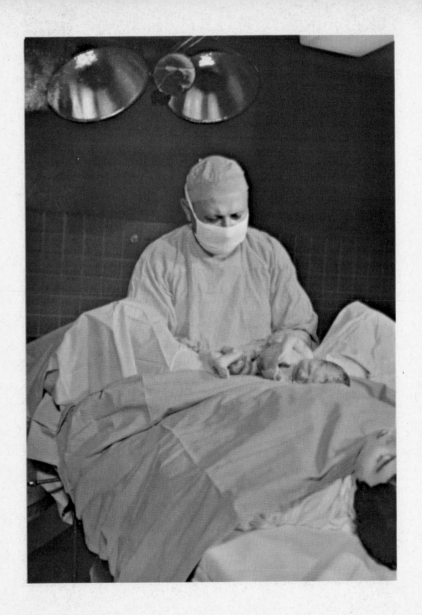

Then the baby is placed on its mother's abdomen.

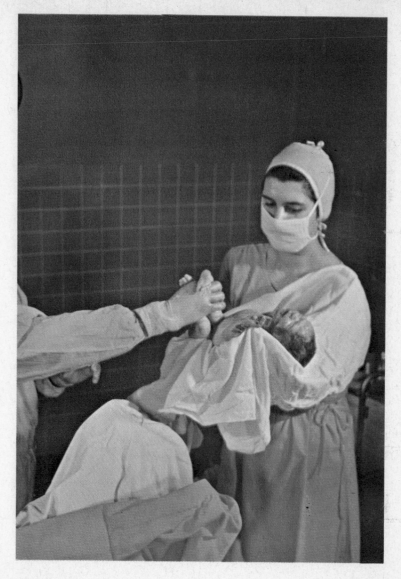

The doctor hands the new arrival to the nurse who places the infant in the bassinet.

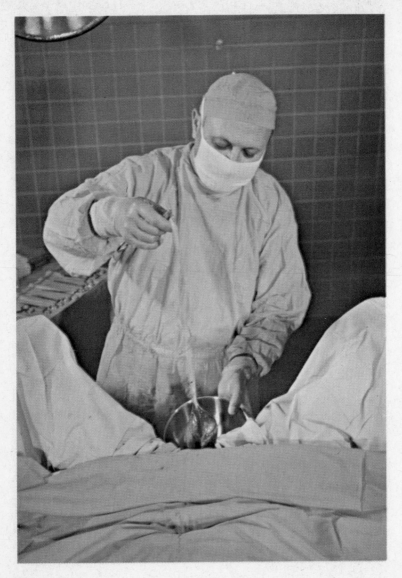

Now the afterbirth is delivered. The small incision used earlier to aid delivery is repaired and the normal anatomy is restored.

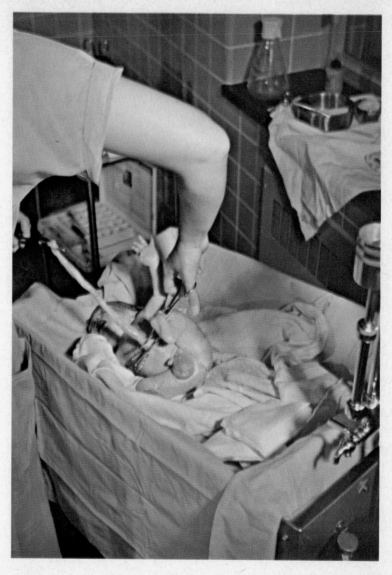

The baby's cord is tied and drops are placed in its eyes to prevent infection.

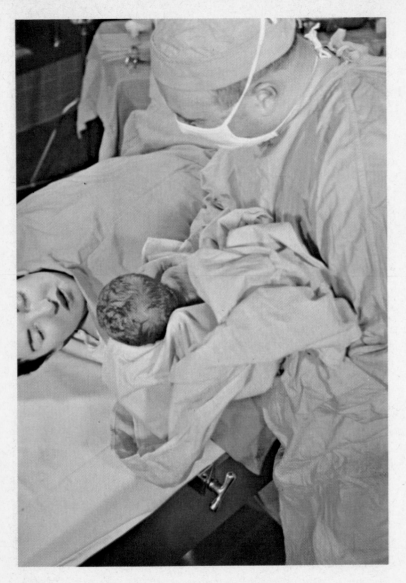

Betsy gets her first good look at her baby and decides that every bit of the previous nine months of waiting have been worth it.

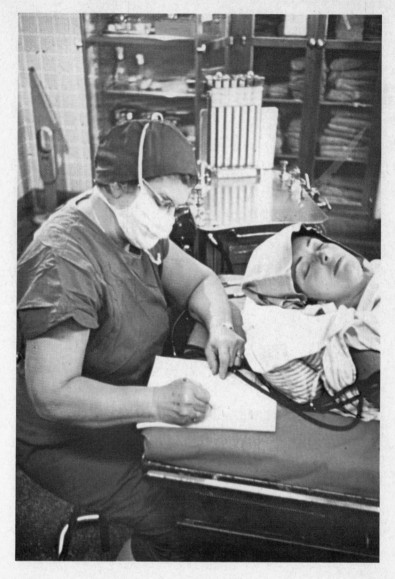

A nurse records the time of the baby's birth along with other pertinent information concerning the delivery.

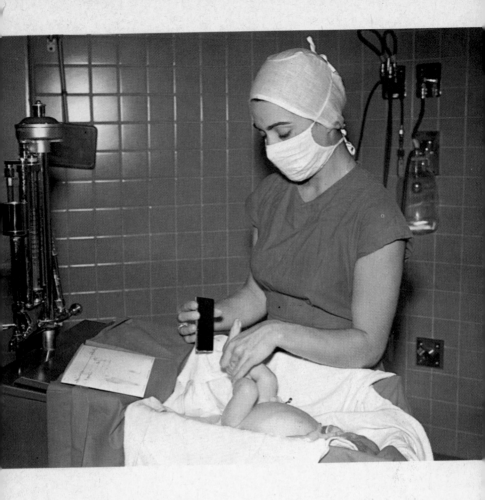

The baby's footprint is indelibly recorded and an identifying band that matches Betsy's is placed on the child.

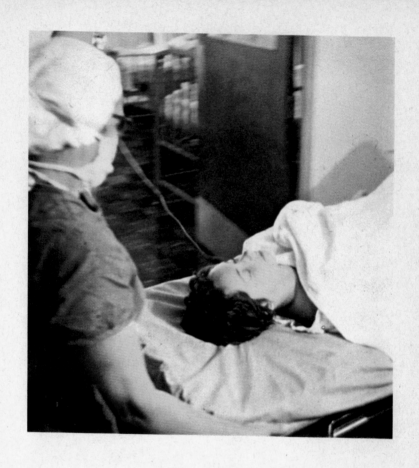

As Betsy leaves the delivery room, the doctor goes to look for Jim.

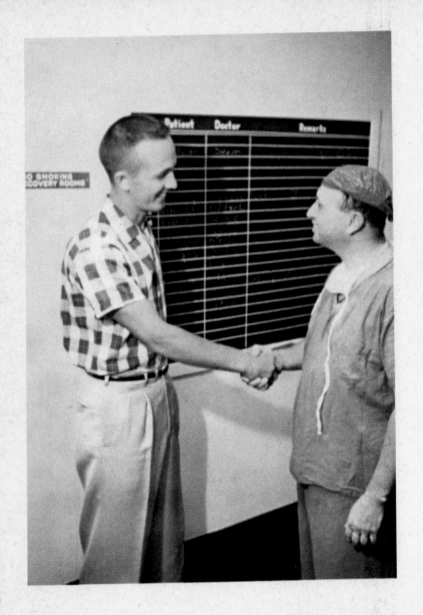

"Well, Jim, congratulations! Betsy is fine and the baby is a beauty."

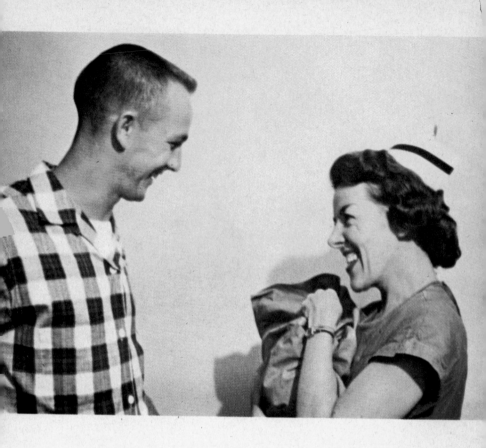

The father of thirty minutes standing is greeted by the nurse with his baby.

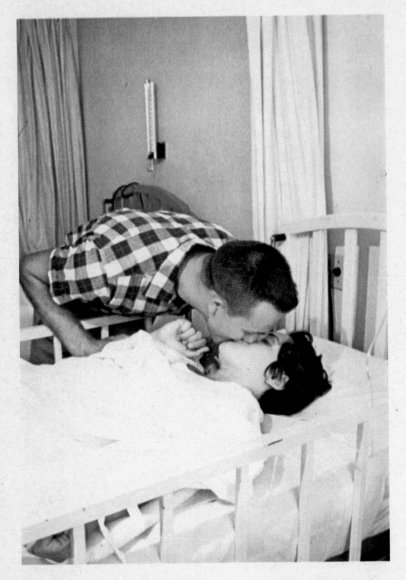

Minutes later he lets Betsy know in no uncertain terms just how wonderful he thinks she is and what a great job she's done.

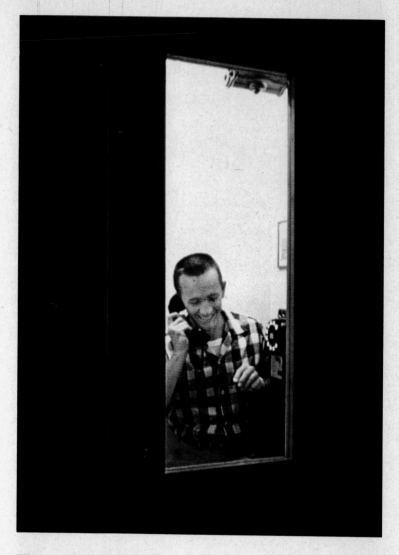

Then, in the tradition of all new fathers, he rushes off to take care of some very important details. "... just what we wanted ... seven pounds, two and three-quarter ounces ... she feels wonderful ... we're both thrilled ..."

Remember

1. Obtain adequate rest.
2. Exercise daily.
3. Eat balanced diet—lean meat, fruit and vegetables, milk.
4. Restrict salt intake.
5. Take prenatal capsules daily as prescribed.
6. Drink several glasses of water daily.
7. Wear maternity foundation or girdle and proper bra.
8. Wear sensible shoes.
9. Have dentist check teeth.
10. First seven months tub or shower. Last two months shower only.
11. Check with doctor before traveling long distances.
12. Bring urine specimen to office each time.
13. Follow your doctor's instructions.

Caution

1. Avoid fatigue.
2. Avoid strenuous exertion.
3. Avoid fried and fatty foods and rich desserts.
4. Avoid potato chips, pretzels, pickles, olives, luncheon meats or highly seasoned foods.
5. Consult your doctor before taking a long automobile trip.
6. Do not douche.

Call the doctor if:

There is vaginal bleeding or spotting.
The bag of water ruptures.
Regular, recurrent contractions occur.
You have blood or pain with urination.
You have chills or fever.
You have severe constipation.
You swell or gain weight suddenly.
The baby stops moving for more than 24 hours.
There are any problems that worry or bother you.

When you have started into active labor do not eat or drink anything. Call the doctor.

Important Information

Doctor's Name _____

Address _____

Telephone _____

Doctor's Night or
Emergency No. _____

Doctor's Associate _____

Telephone _____

Nurse's Name _____

Telephone _____

Hospital Name _____

Address _____

Telephone _____

Taxi _____

Police _____

Pharmacy _____